Raising a healthy and happy family even as you age:Simple aids on parenting kids

Michael Woods

table of contents

Chapter 1

FAMILY FITNESS AND DIETING

FITNESS\What Is Family Fitness.

The Big Benefits of Family Fitness.

Get Started With a Family Fitness Plan.

Family Fitness, Age by Age.

AllFamily fitness:

exercising and generally living a healthy lifestyle as a group is for every family, big and small, young and elderly, urban and rural. By sharing physical activities and nutritional meals, your family may enhance your health and enjoy your time together. Use active activities, smart foods, kid sports, and more to establish healthy habits for your complete "home team."

- The Big Benefits of Family Fitness

Those behaviors may bring loads of wonderful benefits you probably already know about. Being physically active and eating healthy promotes illness prevention, weight loss or maintenance, stress reduction, enhanced performance at school and work, greater lifespan, and more. 1

As parents, we are role models for our kids, so making family fitness a priority creates a terrific precedent. But we get something out of the bargain too. Role modeling helps keep us responsible for our actions.

It may be incredibly motivating to know your youngster is watching. Keep that in mind if you ever feel bad about spending time on exercise.

For youngsters, being exposed to healthy habits early is a blessing. They are so eager to absorb and retain new knowledge and build excellent habits while they are young. Doing so will assist increase their physical confidence, too. And everyone in the family may benefit from the camaraderie that comes from sharing physical play and family dinners.

Get Started With a Family Fitness Plan:The first step to a fun and successful strategy is a goal. Maybe you're worried about your child's weight or your own. Maybe you've observed your family's routines and pastimes tend to be sedentary instead of active. Maybe you made a goal (for the New Year, a birthday, or back to school) to modify your lifestyle.

Maybe you're planning an active summer trip, or your youngster wants to join a sports team and has to get in shape. Whatever your motivation, there are dozens of methods to get started on increasing your family's health.

Creating a family fitness regimen should not be hard or stressful. What it truly implies is a fresh commitment to bringing more movement to your life. It could help to conceive of it as a problem you confront jointly. Work on giving the message that physical exercise is a pleasurable, healthy habit that makes you feel good, not a duty to be endured. You can accomplish this by:

Ask your kid to teach you: Are they a fantastic skater or a whiz at water polo? Request a lesson! Active youngsters enjoy showing off their skills.

Enjoying exercise: Whether it's a rigorous kickboxing class or a stroll, tell your youngster how you feel once you're done. Energized? Happier? Tired, yet pleased with what you accomplished?

Playing together: Kids love your attention. Take kids to the playground, go outdoors for a game of catch, or have a spontaneous dance party.

Praising effort, not results: Your youngster won't be able to ride a two-wheeler or sink a basket on their first try. To stave off frustration (in both passive and active youngsters), make sure to emphasize how hard they're trying.

Offering positive reinforcement: If your youngster makes a healthy decision, recognize it out loud. When they learn a new ability, film it on video, and display it to friends and family.

Setting a good example: Choose activity over gadgets whenever you can. Walk to the store instead of driving, take the stairs, and shelve the leaf blower in favor of a rake. Even if you're not sporty, you can move!

Don't fall victim to confidence-zappers like employing exercise as punishment, giving food as a reward, or utilizing fear tactics. Instead of, "If you watch too much TV, you'll grow fat and ill," offer something like, "Riding your bike helps make your legs and heart strong."

If they're old enough, speak to your kids about what you're doing and gain their buy-in. What are their favorite healthy snacks? Which exercise class would they prefer to attend at your local community center? What family fitness goal can you strive toward together and how may you reward yourselves?

Look at your calendar and attempt to add just a small amount of action at a time, like 15 minutes, two or three days a week. That may involve walking to school, going for a bike trip, or playing a brief backyard game. Eventually, build up to at least 150 minutes each week per family member.

- Family Fitness, Age by Age:

While all children need daily physical activity, their interests and abilities change as they grow. Know what your kid needs today.

Physical Activity for Preschoolers (Plus: Active Toy Ideas for Little Kids) (Plus: Active Toy Ideas for Little Kids)

Fitness for School-Aged Kids (Plus: Toy Picks) (Plus: Toy Picks)

Fitness for Teens and Tweens (Plus: Toys They Won't Outgrow)

Share Active Play

Ready, set, go! The goal is to discover exercise activities that excite you to keep going. Change things up regularly to avoid sliding into a rut. Look for activities, workouts, and games that you can do together, individually, or both whatever works for your family. To get you started:

22 Playful, Physical Outdoor Activities for Kids

Active Options for Family Game Night

Big Fun With Simple Toys

Easy Exercises for Kids

Fit and Fun Social Activities

Pump Up Playtime With Playground Activities

- All About Youth Sports:

How to Be a Good Sports Parents/Family Fitness for Moms and Dads:

Fitting in exercise is a significant issue for most parents, no matter what your personal circumstances are. Sometimes the hurdles are logistical, sometimes physical, sometimes mental. To overcome them, keep trying until you discover a solution that works.

That may include rearranging your schedule; discovering an unexpected, affordable fitness class or workout opportunity; organizing your house to stimulate exercise; checking out a group fitness class or podcast that inspires you; or fighting to combat fitness backsliding. Once you get into a rhythm, you'll want to focus on staying with a fitness program.

A Word From Verywell

Family fitness is a manner of life, not an overnight fix. Give yourself time and space to make adjustments and create new habits. Slow and steady wins this race, but you can win it. You need the proper attitude and the correct tools, and you can find them right here.

FAMILY DIETING:all Here's you need to know for this plan:

1. Don't miss meals. Each night, check the following day's agenda and pre-plan your food so you're equipped with realistic guidance.
2. Stay hydrated. Fill up a water bottle in the morning and start drinking.
3. Aim to refill (and finish) it several times throughout the day. If you'd want a particular quantity to ingest, split your weight in half and that's the approximate number of fluid ounces you should drink in a day. For example, if you weigh 140 pounds aim for 70 ounces each day.

Organize family meals by giving a "theme" to each night. For example: Meatless Mondays, Taco Tuesdays, "Breakfast for Dinner" Wednesdays, Burger Thursdays , "Pizza, Please!" Fridays, Stir-Fry Saturdays and Slow Cooker Sundays

4. Embrace your slow cooker. Use it twice per week for family dinners.

Create a cache of home-cooked meals in your freezer. Over the weekend, make at least 1 dish that can be doubled or tripled, and then put leftovers into containers and freeze for future meals.

Keep emergency snacks in your luggage at all times.Enjoy limitless quantities of non-starchy vegetables: Like carrots, tomatoes, peppers, celery, cucumbers, etc.) at any point throughout the day.

Eat immune-boosting foods. Include at least one of the following immune boosters every day: bell peppers, citrus fruits, pumpkin seeds, yogurt, sweet potato, carrots, spinach and kale, beans (all sorts) (all varieties).

5. LIMIT ALCOHOL TO AT LEAST THREE DRINKS FROM THE ONES LISTED BELOW.

1. Mug scrambled eggs:Make scrambled eggs using the recipe found here. Serve with 1 slice of whole grain bread and 1 tablespoon whipped butter, jam or piece of fruit.

2. Sweet potato toast with peanut butter and banana:Make sweet potato toast with peanut butter and banana using the recipe found here.

3. Greens-in-a-glass smoothie + eggs:Make smoothie following the recipe provided here. Serve with 1 hard-boiled egg or 4 egg whites.

4. Oatmeal with fruit and nuts:Prepare 1/2 cup dried oats with water. Top with 1/2 cup chopped fruit and 2 tablespoons chopped walnuts. Add an optional sprinkling of cinnamon and 1 tablespoon of maple syrup, honey or sugar.

5. Joy's protein pancakes:Prepare Joy's protein pancakes using the recipe listed here. Serve with 1 optional teaspoon of maple syrup or 1 dollop of low-fat Greek yogurt.

6. Breakfast pizza with fruit:Make morning pizza following the recipe given here. Serve with 1/2 pink grapefruit or 1 orange.

LUNCH:

1. Chicken or fish with vegetables:

For this restaurant choice, purchase 1 house salad appetizer with 1 tablespoon vinaigrette (or swap for shrimp cocktail, grilled calamari, or a cup of soup) (or substitute for shrimp cocktail, grilled calamari, or a cup of soup.) Order fish or skinless chicken cooked grilled, roasted, broiled or poached for a main meal. Add a side of steaming, grilled or roasted vegetables.

2. Dinner leftovers:Eat leftovers from supper on day one.

3. Kitchen sink salad:Top mixed greens with 5 ounces of protein (chicken, turkey, salmon, shrimp or tofu) (chicken, turkey, salmon, shrimp or tofu). Add 1/2 cup beans and unlimited non-starchy vegetables. Dress with 2 tablespoons of vinaigrette.

4. Chicken and vegetable wrap:Wrap 4 ounces grilled chicken breast, spinach leaves and choice vegetables on a whole grain tortilla. Serve with a serving of red pepper spears or other crunchy, simple vegetables.

5. Japanese sushi lunch:Order or make 5 pieces of maki roll or 4 pieces of sushi (bonus points for brown rice) (bonus points for brown rice). Serve with a bowl of miso soup and 1 cup edamame.

6. Open-faced turkey and Swiss sandwich.

SNACKS:

1. Apple and peanut butter

Serve apple with 1 tablespoon peanut butter.

2. Sunflower seeds

Enjoy 1/4 cup sunflower seeds.

3. String cheese and pear

Enjoy 1 stick of string cheese and 1 pear.

4. DIY trail mix

Combine 1/2 cup whole grain cereal, 2 tablespoons of almonds or peanuts and 1 tablespoon raisins or dried cranberries.

DINNER:

1. Pesto pasta and salad:\sServe 1 dish of pesto spaghetti using the recipe described here. You may increase the portion size to 2 servings of the same dish if you use zucchini noodles for regular spaghetti. On the side, have a salad with unlimited non-starchy vegetables topped with 2 tablespoons vinaigrette.

2. Turkey tacos

Make 2 tacos using the recipe found here.

3. Slow cooker oatmeal and side of scrambled eggs

Make 1 serving of slow cooker oatmeal using the recipe found here. Top with 1/2 chopped apple, 2 tablespoons chopped walnuts and 1 teaspoon maple syrup. On the side enjoy 1 scrambled egg and 3 egg whites combined with preferred veggies and 2 tablespoons shredded cheese.

4. Turkey black-bean burgers and sweet potato fries:

Make turkey burgers following the recipe listed here. Serve on a whole grain bun with 1 tablespoon ketchup, 1 teaspoon optional mayo, lettuce, tomato, onions, and pickles. Serve sweet potato fries on the side using the recipe described here.

5. Thin-crust vegetable pizza:

Enjoy 2 slices of any thin-crust veggie pizza (frozen, restaurant or homemade) (frozen, restaurant or homemade). For a homemade version with a sweet potato crust use the recipe found here or this version with a cauliflower crust. On the side, serve a salad with non-starchy veggies and 2 tablespoons vinaigrette.

Chapter 2

HABITS SELF-IMPROVEMENT: Bad habits disrupt your life and hinder you from attaining your objectives. They harm your health - both psychologically and physically. And they squander your time and efforts.

So what do we still do with them? And most importantly, is there anything you can do about it?

I've already talked about the science of how habits form, so now let's focus on the practice of making changes in the real world. How do you eliminate your negative habits and stick to positive ones instead?

I don't have all of the answers, but keep reading and I'll share what I've learned on how to quit a bad habit.

What promotes unhealthy habits?

Most of your poor behaviors are caused by two things...

Stress and boredom.

Most of the time, poor habits are merely a technique of coping with stress and boredom. Everything from chewing your nails to going on a shopping spree to drinking every weekend to squandering time on the internet might be a simple reaction to stress and boredom.

But it doesn't have to be that way. You can educate yourself on new and healthy methods to cope with stress and boredom, which you may then swap instead of your old behaviors.

Of course, sometimes the worry or boredom that appears on the surface is driven by underlying concerns. These topics might be challenging to think about, but if you're serious about making changes then you have to be honest with yourself.

Are there particular ideas or motives that are behind the harmful habits? Is there anything deeper — a fear, an experience, or a limiting belief — that is prompting you to cling to something terrible for you?

Recognizing the origins of your poor behaviors is key to resolving them.

You don't erase a negative habit, you replace it

All of the behaviors that you have right now — good or terrible — are in your life for a purpose. In some ways, these habits benefit you, even if they are unhealthy for you in other ways.

Sometimes the advantage is biological as it is with smoking or medicines. Sometimes it's emotional as it is when you remain in a relationship that is horrible for you. And in many circumstances, your unhealthy habit is a simple technique to deal with stress. For example, chewing your nails, twisting your hair, tapping your foot, or clenching your jaw.

These "benefits" or arguments apply to lesser unhealthy behaviors as well.

For example, reading your email inbox as soon as you switch on your computer could help you feel connected. At the same time glancing at all of those emails undermines your productivity, divides your focus, and overwhelms you with worry. But, it prevents you from feeling like you're "missing out" … and so you do it again. Because negative habits bring some form of value to your life, it's quite tough to just eradicate them. (This is why basic advice like "just quit doing it" seldom works.)

Instead, you need to replace negative behavior with a new one that gives a comparative advantage.

For example, if you smoke when you become anxious, then it's a lousy strategy to "just quit smoking" when that occurs. Instead, you should come up with an alternative strategy to cope with stress and insert that new habit instead of taking a smoke.

In other words, unhealthy behaviors meet specific demands in your life. And for that reason, it's best to replace your unhealthy behaviors with a good action that meets a similar need. If you expect yourself to just cut out harmful habits without replacing them, then you'll have certain requirements that will be unsatisfied and it's going to be hard to keep to a pattern of "just don't do it" for very long.

HOW TO BREAK A NEGATIVE HABIT: Here are some extra suggestions for breaking your bad habits and thinking about the process from a different perspective.

1. Choose an alternative for your problematic behavior. You need to have a strategy ahead of time for how you will behave when you meet the tension or boredom that causes your bad behavior. What are you going to do when you experience the temptation to smoke? (Example: breathing exercises instead.) What are you going to do when Facebook is screaming to you to procrastinate? (Example: write one phrase for work.) Whatever it is and whatever you're dealing with, you need to have a plan for what you will do instead of your negative habit. Cut off as many triggers as possible. If you smoke while you drink, then don't go to the pub. If you consume cookies while they are in the home, then toss them all away. If the first thing you do when you sit on the sofa is pick up the TV remote, then conceal the remote in a closet in a separate room. Make it simpler for yourself to break harmful behaviors by avoiding the things that trigger them.

Right now, your environment makes your bad habits easy and healthy ones harder. Affect your surroundings and you can change the result.

2. Join forces with someone. How frequently do you attempt to diet in private? Or maybe you "quit smoking" ... but you kept it to yourself? (That way no one will see you fail, right?)

Instead, hook up with someone and quit together. The two of you may keep each other responsible and enjoy your accomplishments together. Knowing that someone else expects you to do better is a great drive.

3. Surround yourself with individuals who live the way you want to live. You don't need to forsake your existing pals, but don't underestimate the value of discovering some new ones.

4. Visualize yourself succeeding. See yourself putting away the smokes or purchasing healthier food or getting up early. Whatever the negative habit is that you are attempting to break, envision yourself smashing it, smiling, and enjoying your accomplishment. See yourself establishing a new identity.

You don't need to be someone different, you simply need to return to the old you. So frequently we assume that to stop harmful habits, we need to become a different person. The reality is that you already have it in you to be someone sans your harmful habits. It's quite improbable that you have had these unhealthy behaviors all of your life. You don't need to stop smoking, you simply need to return to being a non–smoker. You don't need to convert into a healthy person, you simply need to return to being healthy. Even if it was years ago, you have already lived without this bad habit, which means you can most definitely do it again.

5. Use the word "but" to combat negative self–talk. One problem with overcoming unhealthy behaviors is that it's easy to condemn yourself for not doing better. Every time you trip up or make a mistake, it's simple to remind yourself how much you stink.

Whenever it occurs, end the phrase with "but"...

"I'm overweight and out of shape, but I might be in shape a few months from now."

"I'm foolish and nobody respects me, but I'm attempting to build a worthwhile skill."

"I'm a failure, but everyone fails sometimes."Plan for failure. We all goof up now and again.

Chapter 3

Build Loving Family Relationships nurturing acceptance and understanding within the family.

One of the primary problems that most families endure is in the area of family connections. Everyone encounters some amount of disagreement among family members, and if we let these disputes go unresolved, they will bring division and bitterness into our family and will reduce our effectiveness for the Lord.

As home-educating parents, we confront the full-time burden of ensuring that our children's spiritual, bodily, and educational needs are satisfied. In the middle of all, it is easy to lose out on fostering meaningful ties that will take them into their adult years. Since there is numerous potential for disagreements, we would want to encourage creating loving relationships inside the family.

- Maintain a Loving Relationship between parents

It is critically crucial that parents have a loving connection with each other. This is one of the nicest things that we can do for our children. When there is turmoil in a marriage, the children will feel insecure.

When parents spend time with each other, developing their connection, resolving problems, investing in one another in practical ways, and enjoying one another, children see that they love and cherish one another. This security will boost the calm and pleasure in the household.

- Win the Hearts of Your Children.

There is nothing of greater importance in this world than the souls of our children. We must have the hearts of our children to influence them for the Lord and guide them in His ways.

Winning the heart of a kid is a unique process for each child, based on his age, maturity, personality, and interests. It generally starts with the parents' commitment to concentrate on doing whatever it takes to develop a deep, God-honoring connection with him.

To have won a child's heart is to have openness with him in which he feels safe in expressing his thoughts, ideas, and ambitions with the parents, being certain that he will be cherished and welcomed. Through this connection of whole-hearted trust and friendship, the parents will be able to teach and encourage their kid to develop a relationship with God and will impact him as he makes choices in life.

Access to the heart offers access to every area of life. It takes an effort to win children's hearts, and it does not always come easily. God will grant insight into this process if we ask. Once we have their hearts, they will comply out of a love connection. Whoever has the heart of a kid will have his life and loyalty—whether it is his parents, friends, or others. Valuing our children, embracing them, and understanding them is crucial to gaining their hearts.

- Accepting Your Children.

As parents, we need to embrace our children as God has loved them and allow Him to love them through us. At times every one of us is unlovable, yet God nevertheless loves us unconditionally. God's display of love should be our model for loving our children unconditionally.

Children need to know that their parents are thankful for them and that they are a crucial part of the family. Showing unconditional love and acceptance for them consistently are crucial for preserving their hearts. If we fail to accomplish this, the children will go to someone else for approval. The idea is for the children to have Mom and Dad be their finest earthly providers of love and support.

There is a significant advantage to praising and complimenting our children regularly. It has been claimed that we should praise someone fifteen times for every time that we offer them correction. Praise fosters an environment of love, excitement, and acceptance. Children crave the praise of their parents. They naturally desire to satisfy them and acquire their approval. Mom and Dad should be their greatest admirers and encouragers!

- Understanding Your Children: We may get to understand our children by listening to them. We must provide full attention to them when they communicate with us.

When we talk to our children, we need to ask ourselves, "Do I smile at them and establish eye contact with them? Am I open to what they have to say? Do they feel that they can express their feelings with me without having me judge them?" Effective parenting needs effective listening abilities, which will promote increased comprehension.It is easy for parents to think ahead of their children and predict what they will say or ask. How many times do we already have our minds made up when our children make a request? "Can we purchase a...?" "No!" Our children need to know that we appreciate their thoughts and perspectives. We do not want to give kids a chance to remark, "My parents simply do not understand." When this occurs, barriers will begin to build up in our relationships.

We have found it beneficial to learn about our children's birth-order inclinations, spiritual talents, love languages, and personality kinds. Studying each of these areas lets us experience life from their viewpoint and learn how they approach certain events.

Chapter 4

Spending quality time with your family is crucial. It not only brings everyone closer together, but it's also helpful for good kid development. With the number of hours that have been added to the usual work week, it may be tough to obtain the quality time your family needs and that can lead to an unhappy home.

Additionally, it appears like the family time has been a lot more costly recently since everything from supper and a concert, to visiting your local theme park has increased substantially in price. With that being stated, many families are seeking free or low-cost activities to do that may make spending valuable family time that much more exciting.

If you are seeking fun and exciting activities to do with your family that won't cost a lot of money, stay reading as the childcare professionals at EduCare Nurseries are going to offer some of their favorite methods to spend quality time with your family at zero cost.

Let's get started:

4 essential ways to Spend Quality Time With Your Family At Zero Cost

Work Together - take on a domestic project as a family. Not only will this get more things done on your to-do list, but it will teach your children some new skills while increasing their self-confidence and teaching them the importance of taking care of the items they own. Some nice suggestions might include painting a room, working in the yard, or basic house maintenance.

PLAY TOGETHER - children appreciate the feeling of success they receive from helping around the home, but they love to play much more. Make playtime even more entertaining by making it a family affair. Whether playing outdoors in the yard or having a family game night with your favorite board games, playing together as a family is both fun and free and may be instructive as well.

EXERCISES TOGETHER - exercise is crucial as it may keep us healthy, fit, and active. Our children learn from our example and if we teach them the value of exercising daily, they will follow healthy behaviors for the rest of their life. Another advantage of exercising together as a family is that it doesn't cost anything

COOK TOGETHER - A good way to get the family together for some quality time is to plan and cook a meal together. Children enjoy cooking and there are various jobs in the kitchen that even younger children may accomplish. You have to prepare supper anyhow, so why not make it a family activity? You may try out a new dish or cuisine that your family hasn't tasted before.